Thyro

How to improve and cure thyroid disorders, lose weight, and improve metabolism with the help of food!

Table of Contents

Introduction   iii

Chapter 1: Thyroid Disorders   1

Chapter 2: Diagnosis and Treatments   9

Chapter 3: Thyroid Issues and Weight Gain   13

Chapter 4: Vital Nutrients   15

Chapter 5: Natural Thyroid Solutions and Tips   21

Chapter 6: Thyroid-Friendly Recipes   34

Introduction

I want to thank you and congratulate you for downloading the book, *"Thyroid Diet: How to Improve and Cure Thyroid Disorders, Lose Weight, and Improve Metabolism with the Help of Food."*

This book contains helpful information about thyroid disorders, and how to improve them with diet.

You will soon discover how the thyroid functions, and the effect it has on your health. You will learn about the many different disorders that can afflict the thyroid, why they occur, and also how to treat them!

This book also includes tips and techniques to help you improve and potentially cure your thyroid disorder through diet! Luckily most thyroid disorders are easily treated.

As this book explains, your diet plays a huge role in regulating thyroid function and keeping your thyroid healthy. Whether you have a thyroid disorder or not, the information provided within will help you to make positive dietary changes, and improve your overall thyroid health!

Thanks again for downloading this book, I hope you enjoy it!

Chapter 1: Thyroid Disorders

Thyroid disorders are conditions that affect the thyroid gland. The thyroid gland is a butterfly-shaped gland located at the front of the neck above the trachea—or windpipe—and directly beneath the Adam's apple. It is comprised of two halves, also called lobes. The two halves are attached together by the isthmus, which is a band of thyroid tissue.

The thyroid produces vital hormones that manage bodily functions such as the way your body consumes oxygen and produces heat. Its main role, however, is to regulate your metabolism—the body's ability to break down food and convert it to energy. It is an essential component of the endocrine system, which is the collection of glands that secretes hormones directly into the circulatory system. In turn, the circulatory system carries these hormones to the organs of the body. Other parts of the endocrine system include the pituitary gland, thymus, and pancreas.

The thyroid releases two main hormones: T3 (tri-iodothyronine) and T4 (thyroxine). A normally functioning thyroid produces about 80% T4 hormones and 20% T3 hormones. While T4 is the primary hormone produced by the thyroid gland, T3 is the strongest and most active of the two. The thyroid also produces calcitonin, which is a hormone that has the ability to lower calcium levels in the blood. These hormones control body temperature, maintain the rate at which the body uses fats and carbohydrates, regulate protein production, and influence heart rate. The hypothalamus and pituitary gland control the rate at which T3, T4, and calcitonin are produced and released.

The process begins when the hypothalamus signals the pituitary gland to produce a hormone called TSH, or thyroid-stimulating hormone. The amount of TSH the pituitary gland releases depends on the amount of T3 and T4 hormones in the blood. In turn, the thyroid gland controls its production of hormones based on the amount of TSH received from the pituitary gland.

Thyroid disorders are relatively common and can develop at any age. The roots of diseases and disorders of the thyroid gland can be traced back to a variety of causes such as dietary deficiency and injury. However, in most cases, thyroid diseases and disorders stem from abnormal thyroid growth, thyroid cancer, nodules within the thyroid, and an overproduction or underproduction of thyroid hormones.

The following are some common thyroid conditions, which affect either the function of the thyroid or its structure:

Hyperthyroidism

This is a thyroid disorder caused by an excess of T3 and T4 hormones. In this case, the thyroid is overactive, causing the body's processes to speed up. Symptoms associated with hyperthyroidism include anxiety, irregular heartbeat, excessive sweating, hand tremors, weight loss, and mood swings. In some cases, the disorder gives rise to the formation of a goiter.

The most common cause of hyperthyroidism is an autoimmune disorder called Grave's disease. This disease causes the production of an antibody called thyroid-stimulating immunoglobulin, or TSI by the immune system. This antibody goes haywire and mistakenly attacks the thyroid gland, causing it to produce an excess amount of T4. This overstimulation causes the thyroid to enlarge.

Multinodular goiters are also known to bring about hyperthyroidism. These lumps within the thyroid cause the gland to produce excessive amounts of hormones. Thyroiditis that results from a viral infection may also cause hyperthyroidism, though temporarily. Also, an excessive intake of iodine may cause an overproduction of thyroid hormones.

Hyperthyroidism is readily treated with anti-thyroid medications that inhibit the production of thyroid hormones. An alternative treatment method is to undergo radioactive iodine therapy, which seeks to damage the cells that are responsible for producing thyroid hormones. Beta-blockers that hinder the effects of thyroid hormones on the body—hand tremors, frequent bowel movements, and irregular heart rate, to name a few—are usually taken together with these treatments.

Hypothyroidism

This thyroid disorder is the polar opposite of hyperthyroidism. It is caused by a shortage of thyroid hormones. Unlike hyperthyroidism, *hypo*thyroidism is characterized by an underactive thyroid. It disturbs the normal balance of chemical reactions in the body.

Hypothyroidism symptoms vary depending on the severity of the thyroid hormone shortage. Symptoms include unexplained weight gain, constipation, elevated blood cholesterol levels, joint pain, fatigue, and increased sensitivity to the cold. An enlarged thyroid gland usually arises from hypothyroidism due to the constant stimulation of the thyroid to release more hormones. Furthermore, one may become depressed and forgetful, and thought processes may slow.

If hypothyroidism is left untreated, it may lead to myxedema—a rare form of advanced hypothyroidism. Unlike hypothyroidism, myxedema is usually life-threatening. Unresponsiveness and coma have been documented in patients suffering from myxedema. In severe cases, myxedema can be fatal.

Various factors are known to cause hypothyroidism. Autoimmune diseases produce antibodies in the body that attack normal tissues as well as the thyroid gland. Hyperthyroidism treatments that involve anti-thyroid medications and radioactive iodine may also result in permanent hypothyroidism. Babies born with a congenital disease that leaves them with no thyroid gland or a defective thyroid usually results in a hormone deficiency, thus bringing about hypothyroidism. Iodine deficiency may also result in hypothyroidism.

Goiter

A goiter is an abnormal enlargement of the thyroid gland. It may be a temporary condition that heals itself over time, but in some cases, a goiter is a symptom of another thyroid condition that is severe and requires medical intervention.

Goiters occur when the thyroid gland produces either too much or too little of important hormones—hyperthyroidism and hypothyroidism, respectively. In rare cases, a goiter arises when the pituitary gland—a fellow gland of the endocrine system—stimulates thyroid growth in order to boost hormone production.

A sporadic goiter is another form of abnormal thyroid enlargement. This type of goiter can arise from a diet that includes an excess of goiter-promoting and hormone-inhibiting foods such as cabbage, peanuts, soybeans, and peaches. These foods inhibit the production of thyroid hormones.

Goiters are typically painless, but large goiters may be uncomfortable as they cause coughing and make it difficult to swallow and breathe. Unlike large goiters, small goiters do not usually cause any symptoms. Some common symptoms of a goiter include a visible swelling at the base of the neck, hoarseness, coughing, difficulty swallowing, difficulty breathing, and a tight feeling in the throat.

Iodine deficiency is the most common cause of goiters. Iodine is an indispensable tool in the production of thyroid hormones and is primarily found in seawater. When one is iodine deficient, they may develop a goiter when their thyroid enlarges in an effort to obtain more iodine. Iodine deficiency is made worse when one consumes high quantities of hormone-inhibiting foods.

Several diseases can also give rise to goiters. Grave's disease and Hashimoto's disease are both autoimmune diseases that cause the immune system to attack the thyroid gland. In Hashimoto's disease, this attack results in the production of a lesser amount of thyroid hormone. The thyroid gland enlarges when it senses a low hormone level, causing the pituitary gland to produce more TSH in order to stimulate the thyroid.

Pregnancy may also trigger a goiter. Human chorionic gonadotropin, or hCG—a hormone produced during pregnancy--may cause a slight enlargement of the thyroid gland. Nodules, thyroid cancer, and thyroiditis are also known to cause goiters and will be discussed in more detail later.

While goiters can affect anyone, there are several factors that put one at more risk for developing a goiter. Females are more prone to developing thyroid disorders, thus, they are more likely to develop goiters. Goiters are also likely to occur during pregnancy or menopause. A family history of thyroid diseases and disorders also puts one at a higher risk for developing goiter. Studies have shown that taking lithium and undergoing radiation treatments also increase one's risk of goiter.

Thyroid Nodules

These are solid or fluid-filled lumps that develop within the thyroid. Most thyroid nodules are not serious and do not cause any signs or symptoms. In some cases, however, thyroid nodules grow large enough to be visible as a swelling at the base of the neck and press on the windpipe, causing shortness of breath or difficulty swallowing.

In some cases, thyroid nodules can cause symptoms when they produce an excess of T4 hormones. This occurrence may lead to hyperthyroidism and cause symptoms such as heart palpitations, intolerance to heat, unexplained weight loss, and tremors. While most thyroid nodules are benign, some thyroid nodules are cancerous.

Iodine deficiency can cause the development and growth of nodules in the thyroid gland. An overgrowth of normal thyroid tissue can also cause thyroid nodules to develop, as well as lead to hyperthyroidism. Cysts—or fluid-filled cavities—within the thyroid gland are another cause. Recurrent bouts of thyroid inflammation, Hashimoto's disease, and thyroid cancer often give rise to thyroid nodules.

Thyroiditis

This disease is defined as an inflammation of the thyroid gland. There are several types of thyroiditis, each of them differing in their treatment methods.

The most common type of thyroiditis is Hashimoto's thyroiditis, also known as lymphocytic thyroiditis. The disease is named after Hakaru Hashimoto, a Japanese physician who first described it in 1912. Hashimoto's thyroiditis almost always causes the thyroid gland to swell. Sometimes, only one lobe of the thyroid becomes visibly enlarged. During the course of this disease, the thyroid cells inefficiently convert iodine into thyroid hormones, therefore, the cells compensate for this incompetence by increasing in size. Thyroiditis results in hypothyroidism when the thyroid fails to produce T4 hormones.

Treatment for thyroiditis generally begins with thyroid hormone replacement, which can either prevent the onset of hypothyroidism or remedy it. This treatment also prevents abnormal thyroid enlargement.

Less common than Hashimoto's thyroiditis is De Quervain's thyroiditis, which is also known as subacute thyroiditis. This type of thyroiditis is marked by a rapid enlargement of the thyroid gland, and is accompanied by pain or tenderness. When the thyroid excretes hormones into the bloodstream, it results in hyperthyroidism, which usually corrects itself over a period of several weeks.

De Quervain's thyroiditis is characteristically accompanied by fever. The disease is usually treated with bed rest and over-the-counter anti-inflammatory medications. The thyroid gland usually returns to normal after just several weeks.

The final type of thyroiditis is silent thyroiditis. This disease is uncommon and was not recognized until the 1970s. Silent thyroiditis resembles both Hashimoto's and De Quervain's thyroiditis in equal parts. It typically affects pregnant women. In most cases, the disease requires no treatment as it remedies itself over a period of a few weeks. Some cases of silent thyroiditis, however, have resulted in permanent hypothyroidism.

Thyroid Cancer

Thyroid cancer is uncommon and is characterized by a growth of abnormal cells in the thyroid gland. Those who have thyroid cancer do well because the cancer is usually discovered early on. The sooner treatment starts, the better one's chances of recovery become. Symptoms associated with thyroid cancer include an atypical enlargement of the thyroid gland, pain in the neck or ears, breathing difficulties, a frequent cough that is unrelated to a cold, and hoarseness of the voice.

The cause of thyroid cancer is difficult to pinpoint, but research has shown that, like other cancers, changes in the cell's DNA may be responsible. Those who have been exposed to radiation have the highest risk of developing thyroid cancer. While dental X-rays do not increase one's likelihood of developing thyroid cancer, those who have underwent radiation treatments of the head, neck, or chest are at an increased risk of thyroid cancer.

Thyroid cancer is diagnosed through a biopsy—a procedure in which a tiny piece of tissue is removed and analyzed—of the thyroid gland. The onset of thyroid cancer cannot be prevented. Unlike other cancers, thyroid cancer does not typically require chemotherapy. It is often treated by a combination of surgery and radioactive iodine.

Medullary thyroid cancer, or MTC, is a rare type of thyroid cancer that runs in families. Taking a genetic test will enable one to find out if they are at a risk of developing MTC. If the genetic test is positive, they may opt to undergo surgery to remove the thyroid gland in order to reduce the risk of developing thyroid cancer in the future.

Chapter 2: Diagnosis and Treatments

Diagnosing Thyroid Disorders

Sometimes, physical examinations and a thorough look at family medical backgrounds are not enough to diagnose a thyroid disorder or disease. Oftentimes, patients must undergo specialized tests for diagnosis.

Blood Tests

Blood tests determine the levels of T3, T4, and thyroid-stimulating hormones in the body. They are also used to detect any antibodies against thyroid tissue that may be present in the body.

Ultrasound

When thyroid nodules or enlargement are suspected, imaging tests are commonly used. An ultrasound enables a physician to study and visualize the consistency of a patient's thyroid tissue. While an ultrasound examination can easily recognize enlargement, cysts, or nodules within the thyroid gland, it cannot distinguish a benign growth from a malignant one.

Thyroid Scans Using Radioactive Iodine

Thyroid scans are used to evaluate nodule function in the thyroid gland. Since the thyroid is the only gland in the body that utilizes iodine, it takes up the iodine when radioactively labeled iodine is introduced to it.

Thyroid scans using radioactive iodine shows the uptake of radioactive iodine by normal thyroid tissue. Nodules that are producing an excessive amount of thyroid hormones will show an increased uptake of iodine, and are referred to as "hot" nodules. Those that are referred to as "cold" nodules represent nodules with decreased iodine uptake. In some cases, "cold" nodules are a sign of cancer.

Fine Needle Aspiration Biopsy (FNAP)

Fine needle aspiration biopsy for thyroids is a procedure that entails the removal of a small sample of cells or tissue from the thyroid gland to be examined by a pathologist. FNAP is designed to rule out cancer in a thyroid nodule. It requires the insertion of a long, thin needle to withdraw a sample of cells from the thyroid gland.

Treating Thyroid Disorders

Treatment for thyroid disorders is readily available in the form of medications and surgery. The treatment method varies from case to case, taking a number of factors into careful consideration such as the particular disorder of the thyroid and the severity of the case.

Thyroid Medications

In cases of hypothyroidism and hyperthyroidism, medications to regulate thyroid function are typically prescribed. Patients with hypothyroidism are given medications designed to replace the missing thyroid hormones through the consumption of synthetic thyroid hormone in pill form.

Patients with hyperthyroidism, however, are given anti-thyroid medications to decrease the production of thyroid hormones or inhibit its release from the thyroid gland. Medications designed to relieve the symptoms of hyperthyroidism such as rapid heart rate are also available.

Thyroid Hormone Replacement Therapy

This treatment is designed to compensate for the lack of hormones secreted by the thyroid. In most cases of hypothyroidism, patients are required to take a daily dose of an oral pill of T4 hormone for the rest of their lives.

Radioactive Iodine

This is a treatment method available to patients suffering from hyperthyroidism. Radioactive iodine is designed to gradually shrink the thyroid gland, thus ultimately destroying the gland. Radioactive iodine differs from anti-thyroid medications in that it offers a permanent and more reliable cure for hyperthyroidism. Radioactive iodine ablation is the total destruction of the thyroid gland. In some cases, this treatment is necessary.

Radioactive iodine is obtainable as an oral capsule, thus eliminating the need for hospitalization. Drinking a large amount of fluid induces the release of the radioactive iodine through the urine. Since radioactive iodine only affects the thyroid gland, radiation exposure to the rest of the body's cells is virtually impossible. Once the cells in the thyroid gland absorb the radioactive iodine, they are destroyed indefinitely. The treatment may take several months before the medication completely destroys the thyroid gland. Most patients require only one dose of radioactive iodine to cure their hyperthyroidism, but in some cases, a second dose is required.

All medications are accompanied by side effects, so it is natural that radioactive iodine comes with side effects, too. Common side effects associated with radioactive iodine treatment are nausea, swollen salivary glands, and a metallic taste in the mouth. Ironically, another side effect of this treatment is hypothyroidism. This is because the radioactive iodine destroys a large amount of thyroid cells, resulting in the thyroid's inability to produce a sufficient amount of hormones. In any case, hypothyroidism is much easier to treat than hyperthyroidism.

Thyroid Surgery

Patients undergo thyroid surgery to remove a large goiter or overactive nodules within the thyroid gland. In cases of thyroid cancer, surgery is necessary. If surgery results in the removal of the entire thyroid gland, the patient is required to take synthetic thyroid hormone for life.

The Outlook for Thyroid Disorders

Thyroid disorders are well-managed with the proper medical treatment. In most cases, thyroid disorders are not life-threatening. Some thyroid conditions benefit greatly from surgery, but most conditions are readily controlled by medications. The prognosis for patients with thyroid cancer is good as well.

Chapter 3: Thyroid Issues and Weight Gain

As mentioned in the previous chapters, the thyroid is directly linked to metabolism. In essence, thyroid hormones regulate calorie consumption. Therefore, the gland often influences one's weight.

Many suffering from thyroid disorders—specifically hypothyroidism—complain about a sudden unexpected weight gain. It comes with the territory. The tiniest thyroid imbalance has the power to cause weight gain and other unpleasant symptoms.

Unexpected weight gain followed by difficulty losing extra weight is a telltale sign of hypothyroidism. This is because an underactive thyroid tends to cause an extremely low basal metabolic rate. Hypothyroidism causes your metabolism—the rate at which your body uses nutrients—to slow down. Unexplained weight gain can usually be explained by slow metabolism.

The most effective way to avoid weight gain when you are suffering from hypothyroidism is to regularly observe good nutrition and supplementation. This starts with an appropriate intake of nutrients.

It is important to consume whole foods for optimal nutrition along with a high-quality multivitamin-mineral supplement. A proper intake of iodine, selenium, zinc, copper, and iron promotes thyroid health.

It is also important to eat breakfast within one hour of waking, and to eat balanced meals at regular intervals. Believe it or not, skipping meals is actually detrimental to your thyroid. Missing a meal or a snack puts a strain on thyroid function.

Protein should be included in every meal. In addition, fiber must also be incorporated into breakfast and lunch. Fiber is not only found in grains, but in fruits and vegetables too. It is advisable to eliminate alcohol, junk food, gluten, and sugar from your diet completely as these ingredients tend to interfere with healthy thyroid function.

A balance of good nutrition and supplemental proteins is the only way to furnish the thyroid with the support it needs to strengthen metabolic functioning and lose weight. Observing an optimal diet is crucial in the prevention of additional symptoms associated with thyroid imbalance.

Chapter 4: Vital Nutrients

Thyroid disorders result in one of three possible outcomes: temporary imbalance; lifelong thyroid imbalance; or more severe, often irreversible thyroid conditions.

Fortunately, there are various ways to improve thyroid health easily and naturally by making the most of food and vital nutrients to promote proper thyroid performance. Your dietary habits actually impact your thyroid gland either positively or negatively. The essential nutrients that the thyroid requires are readily accessible in many foods and dietary supplements.

The following list contains and explains the vitamins and minerals that the thyroid needs in order to function:

Iodine

Iodine is essential for thyroid hormone production. Without it, the thyroid would lack the fundamental building blocks it requires to produce the hormones needed to sustain the body. Since the body does not naturally produce iodine, it is imperative to consume iodine-rich foods. An insubstantial amount of iodine in the thyroid results in a shortage of thyroid hormones.

Iodine is primarily found in seawater, soil, and seaweed. Those living inland are typically iodine deficient. In regions such as North America, however, iodine is added to table salt, thus eliminating cases of iodine deficiency among its population. Approximately 40% of the world's population is currently at risk of iodine deficiency.

You can maintain adequate iodine in your diet by eating foods high in iodine. While food labels do not generally list the amount of iodine in foods, dairy products and saltwater fish are usually good sources of iodine. Meat, some breads, eggs, shellfish, and soy sauce also contain iodine. Because it is difficult to identify sources of iodine, multivitamins containing iodine are available.

Although iodine is essential to your diet and plays a key role in preventing thyroid imbalances, excessive iodine intake can cause problems. Large doses of iodine are especially harmful to those who already suffer from thyroid conditions by bringing about hypothyroidism or worsening their hyperthyroid condition. It is crucial to know the appropriate daily intake of iodine to avoid health complications.

Selenium

Selenium is another critical element you should be introducing to your diet. It is a naturally-occurring mineral in soil, water, and some foods. Its antioxidant properties protect cells from damage. Metabolic processes in the human body depend on selenium to operate.

Selenium deficiency has been linked to cancer. Proteins containing selenium assist in the regulation of hormone synthesis, and are responsible for converting T4 into the T3 hormone. T4 hormone only becomes active when it is converted to T3. Furthermore, enzymes containing selenium protect the thyroid during stress by cleansing the gland of oxidative and chemical stress.

These selenium-containing proteins and enzymes help regulate metabolism. They also help maintain suitable levels of thyroid hormones in the organs, blood, and tissues of the body. Also, selenium helps regulate and recycle the body's supply of iodine. Selenium and iodine work arm-in-arm to maintain operational thyroid function. Studies show that a deficiency of both iodine and selenium can worsen thyroid conditions more than a deficiency of iodine alone.

Like iodine, selenium deficiency has strong ties to thyroid imbalances. Selenium is available as a supplement, but the mineral is easily accessible through meats such as tuna, salmon, turkey, lamb, scallops, beef, and chicken. Mushrooms, asparagus, flaxseeds, Brazil nuts, and tofu are also good sources of selenium. It is important to remember that whole foods are the best sources of selenium. The mineral is usually destroyed in foods that are processed.

Selenium does not have any side effects when taken at normal doses. Selenium overdose, however, is known to cause nausea, fever, bad breath, and problems in organs like the heart, liver, and kidney. An excessive intake of selenium supplements puts one at a high risk for developing skin cancer.

Zinc

Zinc is a vital trace element for all living things. It is responsible for maintaining various biological processes and plays a key role in over 300 enzymes in the body. This trace element is required for thyroid hormone synthesis. It is also required for the production of the T3 hormone. Zinc deficiency causes T3, T4, and TSH hormone levels to drop, resulting in thyroid imbalance.

Zinc is primarily introduced to the diet through food. A balanced diet is the best way to provide the body with a sufficient amount of zinc. Oysters, red meat, cereals, poultry, and dairy products are great sources of zinc. Furthermore, zinc supplements and multivitamins containing zinc are available to those with insufficient zinc levels.

Proper doses of zinc must be observed as overexposure may cause low blood pressure, chills, convulsion, and diarrhea.

Iron

The trace element, iron, is vital to good thyroid health. Iron deficiency is a common problem among patients with hypothyroidism. Decreased iron levels cause decreased thyroid function. This deficiency is due to the fact that hypothyroidism typically causes an insufficient amount of stomach acid. This, in turn, results in the malabsorption of iron—the gastrointestinal tract's inability to absorb vital nutrients. Moreover, hypothyroidism tends to cause heavy menstruation which result in more iron loss.

Low levels of iron in the body cause one to have heart palpitations, heat flashes, shortness of breath, and nausea. Supplementing your diet with iron is necessary if your iron levels are low. This can be done by eating foods rich in iron such as liver, lean meats, eggs, leafy vegetables, and whole grain breads and cereals. Cooking in a cast iron skillet also goes a long way in raising your iron levels. Supplemental iron tablets are also available.

Copper

Copper is another trace element the thyroid needs to function well. Copper facilitates the production of TSH while also maintaining T4 production. It stimulates the thyroid and protects the body against excessive T4 in the blood.

Copper imbalance among patients with thyroid disorders not only worsens their condition, but forms a gateway to other health conditions as well. Copper deficiency is known to result in high cholesterol and heart issues among patients with hypothyroidism.

Both copper and zinc are required in sufficient levels to prevent the onset of thyroid conditions and to correct existing thyroid disorders. Zinc supplements tend to deplete copper stores in the body, thus, copper supplements must be taken with zinc.

Natural copper supplementation can be taken by eating foods like sesame seeds, oysters, nuts, lobster, tomatoes, and liver. Overexposure to copper, however, leads to low fertility, heart palpitations, and stomach disorders. Extreme copper toxicity has been linked to kidney and liver damage.

Vitamin A

Vitamin A—commonly known as beta-carotene—deficiency is the most common deficiency worldwide. Vitamin A is crucial for the function of the thyroid hormone receptors. It also stimulates the gene that regulates TSH.

Fruits and vegetables offer an adequate amount of Vitamin A. Some of these include carrots, winter squash, cantaloupe, kale, and sweet potatoes. It is not advisable to supplement with synthetic carotenoids as they can potentially cause health problems.

Antioxidants Vitamin C and Vitamin E

Antioxidants are substances that inhibit cell damage. Vitamins C and E restore thyroid function when the liver is having difficulty detoxifying. These vitamins, along with vitamin A, help the thyroid alleviate stress in an ongoing, daily process.

Vitamin C can be consumed by eating foods such as cauliflower, parsley, peppers, papaya, guava, and strawberries. Peanuts, soybeans, sunflower seeds, and almonds are rich in vitamin E.

B-Vitamins

B-Vitamins are a class of vitamins that are essential for bodily functions such as producing red blood cells and energy production. A deficiency in vitamins B6, B12, or B9 can result in elevated homocysteine—one of twenty amino acids in the body—levels which is closely linked to hypothyroidism. High levels of homocysteine are also associated with stroke, heart attack, and blood clot formation. B9, also known as folate, is important in regulating TSH levels. Vitamins B2, B3, and B6 play a role in the manufacturing of T4 hormone.

Proper intake of micronutrients is crucial as all of these mechanisms are connected. Stress reduces the amount of B-Vitamins in the body. Leafy greens are excellent sources of folate. Poultry, seafood, fortified cereals, and bananas are especially high in vitamin B6. As for vitamin B12, animal foods are the only natural source, but soy products and cereals are fortified with B12, therefore the vitamin is easily accessible.

Asparagine

TSH is made up of substances that include the amino acid called asparagine. Asparagine deficiency can also lead to thyroid disorders, specifically hypothyroidism.

Chapter 5: Natural Thyroid Solutions and Tips

Conventional treatments for thyroid disorders—synthetic thyroid hormone and radioactive iodine—can be supplemented with natural treatments and tips for maximum results. The point of alternative treatments is to target the underlying causes of poor health and resolve them. Sometimes simply treating thyroid symptoms is not enough.

Here are some natural solutions that may help resolve thyroid problems and improve thyroid health:

Avoid Caffeine and Sugar

Caffeine and sugar consumption have negative effects on your health. A high caffeine intake may lead to insomnia, nervousness, nausea, and rapid heartbeat. Excessive caffeine and sugar consumption during pregnancy increases the risk of an early death for the infant or giving birth prematurely.

While it is acceptable to reduce caffeine and sugar intake, it is better to eliminate them completely. Caffeine and sugar have an adverse impact on thyroid health. Consumption of these substances tends to increase metabolism, which may be harmful for someone suffering from thyroid disorders or iodine deficiency.

If you are iodine-deficient while regularly consuming caffeine, your risk for developing thyroid cancer increases. It is a good idea to condition yourself to gradually eliminate caffeine and sugar from your diet.

Exercise Regularly

Those with thyroid conditions can benefit from exercising for just a few minutes each day. Proper exercise can help you fight the symptoms associated with thyroid disorders, lose weight or maintain a healthy weight, and make you feel better overall.

Low-impact aerobics and cardio exercise are recommended for hypothyroid patients. Pilates helps improve your core muscles and ease the back pain that is associated with hypothyroidism. Building muscle helps counter weight gain from an underactive thyroid.

The following lists the best exercises that will enable you to maintain a healthy weight or lose extra pounds:

1. **One-legged dead lift:** Begin by standing on one leg while holding onto something for balance—the back of a sofa or your kitchen counter, for instance. Keep one hand relaxed on your thigh. Push your hips as far back as you can, until your hand touches the ground. Come back up and repeat ten times. If you perform this exercise properly, you feel a burn in the glutes.

2. **Overhead press:** This requires a pair of dumbbells. Raise the dumbbells to shoulder height. Turn your arms so that they are facing forward. Lift the dumbbells up until your elbows are straight before lowering the dumbbells back down to your shoulders.

3. **Squats:** This exercise is fairly simple. Begin by standing up straight, observing good posture. Bend at your hips and knees until you are in a sitting position. Make sure to go down all the way. If performed properly, you will feel the burn in your thighs and glutes.

4. **Push-up:** Place both hands flat on the floor, shoulder width apart. Feet should be stretched back and touching. Bend your elbows and shoulders until your nose is just a few inches away from the ground. If a push-up is too difficult, do the same thing either with your hands on a table or a wall.

5. **Lat pull-down:** Firmly grasp a pull-down bar with an overhand grip. Pull the bar all the way down to your collar bone. The bar should travel as close to your face as possible. It is important to keep your back straight during this exercise with your stomach tight and shoulder blades pulled back.

6. **Rowing:** Sit on the bench of a rowing machine and hold the handle that is attached to the cable. Keeping your back straight, lean back about 10 to 15 degrees. Pull the cable back until it touches your mid-stomach before releasing under control.

Your daily exercise routine should be composed of the six exercises above, or other similar exercises. Complete a few sets of between 8 and 15 repetitions. It is advisable to start slowly; rushing into an exercise routine can injure you. Always consult a medical professional before starting a fitness program. Seeing a personal trainer is also recommended for beginners.

Increase Protein Intake

Proteins are any of a class of nitrogenous organic compounds that consist of large molecules composed of one or more long chains of amino acids. Proteins are an essential part of all living organisms. They serve as structural components of body tissues such as muscle and hair, and as enzymes and antibodies.

Proteins carry thyroid hormones to all your tissues. Including protein at each meal goes a long way in normalizing thyroid function. A diet high in lean protein sources is known to support thyroid health. Conversely, a low-protein diet stresses the body and causes suppression of the thyroid. Furthermore, a diet low in protein reduces the body's response to synthetic thyroid hormone supplements, which lowers overall metabolism further.

It is recommended to incorporate one or two portions of lean protein into each meal. Including protein in your breakfast will stimulate your metabolism for the rest of the day. You should not rely too heavily on vegetables for overall protein intake as doing so lacks sufficient balance. You should not rely too heavily on meat sources either as doing so will likely overwhelm the body with amino acids.

Balancing protein sources is the way to go. For example, it is best to combine a quart of milk with shellfish and potatoes, rather than relying on a single source of protein. Other lean proteins include skinless chicken breast and regulated amounts of lean cuts of pork, lamb, or beef.

Don't Be Afraid of Fats

An insufficient intake of fat and cholesterol is known to worsen hormonal imbalances, including thyroid hormones. Fats are an essential part of a healthy diet. They provide your body with vital fatty acids and fat-soluble vitamins. There are good fats and bad fats; it is just a matter of learning which fats are healthy for you and which ones are not.

You should avoid 'trans-fats' or 'trans-fatty acids' that clog your arteries altogether. Trans-fatty acid is an unsaturated fatty acid that is found in margarines and manufactured cooking oils as a result of the hydrogenation process. Excessive consumption of trans-fatty acids is linked to atherosclerosis—the accumulation of fats and cholesterol in and on the walls of the artery. A diet high in trans-fat can cause strokes, heart disease, and heart attacks. Avoid food containing trans-fat such as commercially-baked pastries and pizza, packaged snack foods, candy bars, fried foods, and margarine.

Saturated fat is also bad for you. It is primarily found in animal food sources such as red meat, the visible fat on meat and chicken, and whole-fat dairy products. Saturated fat triggers a spike in total blood cholesterol levels which increases your risk of diabetes and cardiovascular disease.

Monounsaturated fats and polyunsaturated fats are the healthy fats that are beneficial to your heart, cholesterol levels, and overall health. Both fats are found in a variety of foods and oils. A diet rich in monounsaturated and polyunsaturated fats improves blood cholesterol levels, decreasing your risk of developing heart disease.

Olive oil, peanut butter, sesame oil, and avocados are excellent sources of monounsaturated fats. Polyunsaturated fats can be found in walnuts, safflower oil, flaxseeds, soymilk, and tofu.

Increase Your Nutrient Intake

Nutritional deficiencies put you at a high risk for developing thyroid disorders. The vitamins and minerals listed in Chapter 4 should all be consumed in proper amounts. Here is a list of food sources rich in those vital nutrients:

Iodine: Nori, kelp, oysters, sardines, clams, shrimp, salmon, iodized sea salt, sesame seeds, eggs, lima beans, Swiss chard, asparagus, summer squash, mushrooms, garlic, spinach

Selenium: Brazil nuts, halibut, organ meats, tuna, sunflower seeds, beef, mushrooms, soybeans

Zinc: Lamb, beef, turkey, walnuts, sunflower seeds, oysters, sardines, gingerroot, whole grains, Brazil nuts, pecans, maple syrup, almonds

Copper: Chickpeas, tomato paste, dark chocolate, oysters, lobster, sunflower seeds, beef, crabmeat, shitake mushrooms

Iron: Organ meats, lentils, spinach, clams, oysters, pumpkin seeds, molasses

Vitamin A: Liver, winter squash, sweet potatoes, cantaloupe, asparagus, broccoli, carrots, lettuce, kale, spinach

Vitamin C: Brussels sprouts, cauliflower, broccoli, kale, collard greens, turnips, parsley, Bell peppers, chili peppers, papaya, kiwi, strawberries, guava

Vitamin E: Sunflower seeds, almonds, peanuts, asparagus, liver, whole grains, kale, beans

Vitamin B2: Wild rice, almonds, organ meats, wheat germ, mushrooms, egg yolks, Brewer's yeast

Vitamin B3: Brewer's yeast, white-meat chicken, peanuts, liver, wheat bran, rice bran

Vitamin B6: Trout, salmon, tuna, brown rice, bananas, liver, sunflower seeds, pinto beans, Brewer's yeast, garbanzos, wheat germ, lima beans

Avoid Foods That Disrupt Thyroid Function

Do not eat anything that could interfere with thyroid function if you have an existing thyroid condition. Here are some foods to avoid:

Soy

Soy is a protein derived from soybeans. Consuming an excess amount of soy should be avoided as its plant-based estrogen content tends to suppress thyroid function. Estrogen hinders the release of thyroid hormones which can lead to an underactive thyroid.

Gluten

Gluten is a substance found in cereal grains and wheat. It acts as a glue that holds food together and helps food maintain its shape. Those with existing thyroid conditions are advised to limit their intake of gluten. Gluten is known to irritate the small intestine and hinder the absorption of thyroid hormone replacement medication.

Fatty Foods

It is recommended that you eliminate fried foods from your diet completely if you have an existing thyroid condition. Like gluten, fatty foods inhibit the absorption of thyroid medication. Minimize your intake of fats from sources such as mayonnaise, butter, and margarine.

Sugary Foods

Since slow metabolism is connected to hypothyroidism, you must make careful choices in your diet. Eating foods with a high sugar content makes it easy to gain weight. If you have hypothyroidism, it is a good idea to avoid sugary foods as they are loaded with calories and lack any nutritional value.

Processed Foods

Processed foods are one of the worst things you can put in your diet, especially if you suffer from thyroid imbalance. Foods that have been chemically processed are made solely from refined ingredients and artificial substances like preservatives and colorants. Processed foods are loaded with sodium which is detrimental to those with thyroid problems.

People with an underactive thyroid are at a risk of high blood pressure, and an excess intake of sodium further increases this risk. Processed foods are also high in sugar, fructose corn syrup, and refined carbohydrates, making the hypothyroid consumer gain unnecessary weight. Furthermore, processed foods are low in nutrients and tend to be low in fiber as well.

Some common processed foods include bacon, processed meats, canned vegetables, microwave dinners, cheese, and breakfast cereals. All of these should be avoided as they disrupt thyroid function. Read the *Nutrition Facts* on food labels and packaging and choose the options lowest in sodium. If you have hypothyroidism, you should restrict your sodium intake to 1500 milligrams per day.

Excess Fiber

Fiber is the indigestible component of plant foods that pushes through your digestive system, absorbing water and easing bowel movements. While fiber is essential to your diet, an excessive fiber intake can actually complicate your thyroid treatment. Excessive amounts of dietary fiber from beans, vegetables, legumes, and whole grains has a negative impact on your digestive system and tends to interfere with your body's ability to absorb thyroid hormone replacement medications.

Coffee

Coffee and other sources of caffeine must be eliminated—or at least greatly reduced—from your diet for the sake of proper thyroid function. Coffee tends to inhibit the absorption of thyroid hormone replacement medications.

Alcohol

Excessive alcohol consumption interferes with the regulation of thyroid hormone levels in the body as well as the thyroid's ability to produce T3 and T4 hormones. Studies have shown that alcohol has a toxic effect on the thyroid gland and inhibits the body's ability to use thyroid hormones. If you have hypothyroidism, it is advisable to either drink in moderation or eliminate alcohol from your diet completely.

Be Wary of Goitrogens

Another tip for thyroid health is to be mindful of goitrogens. It is important to learn which foods contain goitrogens—substances that destroy thyroid function by interfering with iodine uptake, which can lead to an abnormal enlargement of the thyroid gland, also referred to as goiter. Goitrogenic foods include pine nuts, cassava, bamboo shoots, and millet. Cruciferous vegetables such as broccoli, cauliflower, and cabbage are also considered to be goitrogenic. It is advisable to steam these vegetables before consuming to eliminate the goitrogens in them.

Introduce More Glutathione into Your Body

Glutathione is the mother of all antioxidants. It is a compound involved as a coenzyme in oxidation-reduction reactions in cells. It is produced naturally in the liver and found in fruits, vegetables, and meats. Glutathione is the most important molecule your body needs to maintain good health and prevent the onset of various diseases.

Because glutathione boosts the immune system, those who suffer from thyroiditis—specifically Hashimoto's thyroiditis and Grave's disease—require sufficient levels of glutathione. Glutathione assists in the healing process of thyroid tissue.

Glutathione is not easily accessible in foods, but there are foods that help the body produce more glutathione naturally. Some of these include asparagus, avocado, peaches, broccoli, squash, grapefruit, and raw eggs. Furthermore, cabbage and cauliflower contain a substance that helps replenish glutathione stores.

Do a Gut Check and Consume Probiotics

A gut check is an evaluation or test of your stomach. About 20% of thyroid function depends on an ample supply of healthy gut bacteria. It is advisable to supplement with probiotics when you have a thyroid disorder.

Probiotics are introduced to the body for their beneficial qualities. Probiotics are considered to be healthy bacteria. Sauerkraut, yogurt, miso soup, kimchi, and pickles are excellent sources of probiotics.

Go on a Heavy Metal Detox

Heavy metal detoxification is the removal of toxic metallic substances from the body such as mercury, lead, and aluminum. These heavy metals accumulate in the body over time, triggering various diseases such as autism, infertility, and thyroid disorders. A heavy metal detox enables you to remove toxic metal contaminants from your body and minimize their impact on your health. It is a six-step procedure that spans a period of several months.

1. **Be particular about fish:** Fish—especially those that have long lifespans—absorb mercury from their environment. Shark, Bluefin tuna, and swordfish all contain high levels of mercury. It is advisable to limit your consumption of these types of fish.

2. **Consider your dental work:** Teeth fillings—especially silver-colored ones—are typically composed of a mixture of mercury. These fillings break down over time. If you have many of these fillings, consider replacing them with tooth-colored resin fillings. Talk to your dentist about this.

3. **Ask for mercury-free vaccines:** Some vaccines contain a mercury-based preservative called thiomersal. It is a controversial organomercury compound that has been removed from most vaccines, but there are still some vaccines out there that contain thiomersal such as flu vaccines. There are mercury-free alternatives, however, but finding them may require some research on your behalf.

4. **Protect yourself against pollution:** Heavy metals are floating in the water and air pollution. Avoid industrial areas and make a point of drinking filtered water. It is also advisable to wear a surgical mask when venturing into congested cities.

5. **Be cautious of old paint:** Lead is a toxic heavy metal and can be found in old paint from the 1970s. Be wary of old structures and places where paint is chipping.

6. **Order a side of cilantro:** Cilantro—also known as coriander—is a natural chelating agent. Chelation is a medical procedure that entails the administration of chelating agents to remove heavy metals from the body. The best part about it is that cilantro does not have to be injected intravenously like other chelating agents. "Cilantro chelation" requires a small amount of fresh cilantro that can be made into a pesto sauce and eaten with pasta or toast. Cilantro should be consumed every day for several weeks.

Lower Your Carbohydrate Intake

Carbohydrates are sugars that your body breaks down to create glucose. In turn, your blood carries the glucose throughout your body. Glucose is the primary source of energy for the brain and other essential cells. Foods high in carbohydrates can be potentially dangerous to thyroid health. Such foods include dried fruits, sweeteners, jams, and cereals.

Lower your intake of sugars and replace them with healthy fats like monounsaturated fats and polyunsaturated fats. Women who consume an excessive amount of carbohydrates show an increase in estrogen levels which affects the thyroid in negative ways. Limit your intake of carbs and replace them with fats that will balance hormone levels such as avocado, grass-fed beef, flaxseeds, and coconut milk.

Avoid BPA

BPA, or bisphenol A, is a carbon-based synthetic compound used in the manufacturing of certain resins and plastics such as water bottles. BPA can leak into food and beverages from plastic containers that are made with BPA. BPA exposure is known to have negative effects on the endocrine system, including the thyroid gland.

Seek out BPA-free products and use alternatives such as glass, porcelain, or stainless steel containers. Avoid eating foods that come from tin cans also, as most of these cans are lined with resin that contains BPA.

Practice Relaxation Exercises

Practicing deep breathing and other techniques that trigger a relaxation response can help improve symptoms associated with thyroid disorders. Meditation and yoga are excellent sources of relaxation. Guided imagery can promote relaxation as well. It is a program of directed thoughts and suggestions that guide your imagination toward a relaxed state.

Get Adequate Sun Exposure

Maintaining vitamin D levels is crucial to thyroid health. Vitamin D promotes healthy immune system function and calcium metabolism. Sunlight is a great source of daily vitamin D as it stimulates the body to produce the vitamin. Fifteen to twenty minutes of unprotected sun exposure twice a day is recommended to maintain an adequate level of vitamin D.

Acupuncture to Correct Thyroid Imbalances

Utilizing both Western and Eastern healing methods provide you with many more options to restore thyroid hormone levels. Including acupuncture in your existing thyroid treatment can be beneficial.

Acupuncture is an ancient Chinese technique that involves pricking the skin with fine needles at certain points of the body. When these needles are inserted, they realign the flow of energy, or *qi*. Acupuncture can help treat thyroid conditions by correcting energy and hormonal imbalances. This is done by stimulating the body's ability to resist illnesses. The best part about acupuncture is that it is free of any adverse side effects.

Chapter 6: Thyroid-Friendly Recipes

Observing a diet rich in nutrients is imperative for any treatment method that seeks to improve thyroid health and repair the thyroid gland. This chapter encompasses various recipes that will enable you to maintain a healthy weight, improve your metabolism, and treat your thyroid disorder.

Thyroid-Friendly Salad

This salad is recommended for those with hypothyroidism who are seeking to maintain good thyroid health.

You will need:

- 1 bunch of kale, coarsely chopped

- 2 carrots, grated

- Red cabbage, chopped into strips

- Cilantro, coarsely chopped

- Sunflower seeds

- 1 tablespoon apple cider vinegar

- 3 tablespoons olive oil

- A pinch of iodized salt

Directions:

1. For the dressing, combine apple cider vinegar, olive oil, and iodized salt. Set aside.

2. For the salad, combine the kale, carrots, cilantro, and red cabbage. Sprinkle over with sunflower seeds and drizzle with salad dressing.

Slow Cooker Vegetarian Chili

The secret to this chili is the butternut squash, which incorporates a layer of flavor and sweetness to the dish.

You will need:

- 2 teaspoons canola oil

- 1 large onion, diced

- 2 stalks celery, diced

- 2 carrots, diced

- 2 cloves garlic, minced

- 1 red bell pepper, diced

- 2 tablespoons chili powder

- 2 teaspoons ground cumin

- ¼ teaspoon red pepper flakes

- 1 can crushed tomatoes

- 3 cans red kidney or black beans, rinsed and drained

- 12 ounces butternut squash, peeled and diced

- 1 cup vegetable stock

Directions:

1. Heat the oil in a pan and sauté the onions, carrots, and celery for 4 minutes. Add the garlic and bell pepper, and sauté for another 2 minutes.

2. Add the spices and cook for 1 minute, stirring constantly. Remove the pan from the heat.

3. Add the vegetables and the remaining ingredients to the slow cooker. Stir to combine. Cover and slow-cook for 6 hours. Serve hot.

Simple Quinoa and Vegetables

This recipe is not only vegetarian, but extremely rich in protein, too. It is easy to prepare and is packed with flavor.

You will need:

- 1 cup quinoa, rinsed

- 2 cups water

- 4 medium carrots, chopped

- 1 zucchini, chopped

- 8 asparagus spears, chopped

- 1 tablespoon rice wine vinegar

- 2 tablespoons olive oil

- 1 tablespoon fresh thyme

- Black pepper and iodized salt to taste

Directions:

1. In a saucepan, bring the water to a boil. Add quinoa and stir. Cover and simmer for 12 minutes, or until the water is absorbed. Once the quinoa is cooked, fluff it with a fork.

2. Steam the vegetables for 3 minutes.

3. For the vinaigrette, whisk together rice wine vinegar and thyme in a small bowl.

4. To assemble, place quinoa on a plate and arrange the vegetables over it. Drizzle over with the vinaigrette.

Caribbean Fish with Mango Salsa

This recipe is sure to blow your taste buds away and provide you with essential nutrients.

You will need:

- 1 egg

- 1/3 cup milk

- 1 cup panko breadcrumbs

- 1 tablespoon dried, unsweetened coconut

- 1 tablespoon olive oil

- 5 tilapia fillets

For the fish spice:

- 1 tablespoon paprika

- 2 teaspoons curry powder

- 2 teaspoons ground cumin

- 1 ½ teaspoon ground allspice

- 1 teaspoon ground ginger

- 1 teaspoon ground coriander

- ¼ teaspoon ground fennel seed

- 1/8 teaspoon cayenne pepper

- ¾ teaspoon iodized salt

- ½ teaspoon ground black pepper

For the mango salsa:

- 1 mango, peeled and diced

- 1 cup pineapple, diced

- ½ red bell pepper, diced

- ½ cup black beans, rinsed and drained (optional)

- ½ red onion, minced

- 3 tablespoons cilantro, coarsely chopped

- Juice of one lime

Directions:

1. In a bowl, mix together all of the spices and set aside.

2. In another bowl, mix together all of the ingredients for the mango salsa. Cover and refrigerate until chilled.

3. Whisk together the egg and milk in a bowl. In a separate bowl, stir together the coconut and panko bread crumbs. Incorporate 1 tablespoon of the spice mix into the coconut and panko mixture.

4. In a skillet, heat olive oil over medium heat. Dip the tilapia fillets into the egg mixture, then press gently into the panko crumb mixture and coat both sides of the fillets. Shake off any loose crumbs, then lay the fillets into the hot oil. Pan-fry until the fish is golden-brown, 3 to 5 minutes per side. Serve with mango salsa.

Sesame Almond Butter Noodles

This dish can be prepared raw or cooked. The sesame noodles are iodine-rich and nearly calorie-free.

You will need:

For the almond butter sauce:

- ¼ cup almond butter

- 1 tablespoon rice vinegar

- 1 tablespoon agave nectar

- 1 tablespoon sesame oil

- ¼ cup tamari

- 1 teaspoon Sriracha

- 1 teaspoon ginger, minced

For the noodles:

- 2 (12-ounce) bags kelp noodles, rinsed and drained

- 1 red bell pepper, cut into thin strips

- 2 medium carrots, julienned

- 3 green onions, thinly sliced

- 2 tablespoons sesame seeds

- ¼ cup cashews

Directions:

1. Whisk together in a small bowl all the ingredients for the almond butter sauce.

2. In a separate large bowl, combine the noodles, bell pepper, and carrots. Add the almond butter sauce and toss to coat evenly. Refrigerate until chilled.

3. Garnish with green onions, cashews, and sesame seeds before serving.

Curried Split Pea Cauliflower Stew

This dish makes use of cauliflower and legumes—good sources of vitamin C and fiber.

You will need:

- 1 1/3 cups yellow split peas, parboiled

- 1 head of cauliflower, sprinkled with 1 tablespoon curry powder and a pinch of sea salt, and roasted in a 400-degree oven for 20 minutes.

- 1 tablespoon coconut oil

- 1 teaspoon mustard seeds

- 1 teaspoon cumin seeds

- 1 large yellow onion, diced

- 1 large carrot, diced

- 1 knob ginger, grated

- 6 cloves garlic, minced

- 2 tablespoons curry powder

- 1 teaspoon ground turmeric

- 2 cups vegetable broth

- 1 (15-ounce) can coconut milk

- 2 teaspoons apple cider vinegar

- 1 teaspoon garam masala

- 1 teaspoon sea salt

- Chopped cilantro for garnish

Directions:

1. Parboil the split peas for roughly 45 minutes. Drain and set aside.

41

2. In a large pot, heat the coconut oil. Cook the mustard seeds and cumin seeds and cover with the lid. The seeds will make a popping sound. When the popping ceases, add the onion and sauté for 4-5 minutes.

3. Add the carrot, garlic, and ginger. Cook for 1 minute. Add the curry powder and turmeric. Cook for 30 seconds, stirring constantly.

4. Add the vegetable broth, parboiled split peas, and coconut milk. Reduce the heat and gently simmer for 15 minutes, stirring occasionally.

5. Add the roasted cauliflower, apple cider vinegar, garam masala, and sea salt. Simmer for another 10 minutes. Serve hot with chopped cilantro for garnish.

Slow Cooker Honey-Garlic Chicken Thighs

A hit with kids and adults alike, this dish requires just a few ingredients from your pantry and refrigerator. It is super easy to make, and best when serve with quinoa, basmati rice, or steamed vegetables.

You will need:

- 4 chicken thighs skinless, deboned

- 1/3 cup honey

- ½ cup ketchup

- ½ cup soy sauce

- 1 tsp dried basil

- 3 cloves garlic, minced

Directions:

1. Arrange the chicken thighs into the bottom of a slow cooker.

2. In a bowl, whisk together the rest of the ingredients and pour over the chicken.

3. Set to low and cook for 6 hours.

Baked Stuffed Pumpkin

Pumpkin is an excellent source of fiber, and its seeds are good sources of protein. This is the perfect dish to prepare during the fall season.

You will need:

- 1 medium pumpkin

- 2 cups cooked brown rice

- 1 cup pecans, coarsely chopped

- 1 ½ cups fresh cranberries

- 1 cup chicken stock

- 2 teaspoons iodized salt

- 2 tablespoons ground flaxseed

- 2 stalks of sage, chopped

- 2 tablespoons olive oil

Directions:

1. Preheat the oven to 400-degrees Fahrenheit.

2. Cut off the top of the pumpkin and scrape out the seeds. (The seeds can be toasted later for a fun and nutritious snack.) Rub the exterior of the pumpkin with olive oil.

3. For the stuffing, combine all the ingredients in a large bowl. Stuff the pumpkin and cover it with the pumpkin top.

4. Place the pumpkin on a tray and bake for 1 hour, or until softened.

Cucumber Avocado Summer Soup

Cucumbers are rich in antioxidants, and avocados are a great source of healthy fats, minerals, and vitamins.

You will need:

- 3 lbs. cucumber, chopped

- 2 avocados, chopped

- ½ bunch fresh mint, chopped

- ½ bunch cilantro, chopped

- 2 cloves garlic, minced

- 2 tablespoons ground cumin

- The zest and juice of 1 lemon

- 1 ½ teaspoons iodized salt

- Extra virgin olive oil and chopped almonds for garnish

Directions:

1. Place the cucumbers, mint, cilantro, cumin, lemon juice and zest, salt, and garlic into a food processor. Process until smooth.

2. Add chunks of avocado and continue blending until the mixture is smooth. Chill for a few hours.

3. Just before serving, drizzle the summer soup with olive oil and sprinkle with almonds.

Quick Zucchini and Anchovy Salad

Here is another recipe that is quick and easy to prepare. Anchovies provide your diet with iron, which is a crucial element for thyroid health. Zucchini, on the other hand, is a great source of vitamin C.

You will need:

- 1 large zucchini, peeled and julienned

- 1 can anchovies or sardines, mashed with a fork

- 1/3 bunch of dill, chopped

- 2 tablespoons olive oil

- Juice of 1 lemon

- Iodized salt to taste

Directions:

1. In a bowl, whisk together the olive oil, lemon juice, and iodized salt.

2. In a separate bowl, mix together the remaining ingredients.

3. Pour the vinaigrette over the salad and toss well.

Almond Bread

A delicious recipe that is gluten-free, low-carb, and protein-rich.

You will need:

- 2 ½ cups almond meal

- 1 ½ teaspoon arrowroot powder

- 1 tablespoon baking powder

- 1 teaspoon iodized salt

- 3 eggs, beaten

- 1 tablespoon honey

- ½ teaspoon apple cider vinegar

Directions:

1. Preheat the oven to 300-degrees Fahrenheit.

2. In a large bowl, mix together the almond meal, arrowroot, baking powder, and iodized salt.

3. In a separate bowl, whisk together the eggs, honey, and vinegar.

4. Stir the wet ingredients into the dry ingredients.

5. Pour the batter into a greased baking dish and bake for 45-55 minutes.

Almond Flour Zucchini Apple Pancakes

This recipe incorporates savory and sweet flavors, and helps you to maintain a healthy blood sugar level. It is perfect for those who are eliminating grains from their diet.

You will need:

- 1 small zucchini, grated

- 1 small apple, grated

- 1 cup almond flour

- ½ teaspoon baking powder

- ½ teaspoon iodized salt

- 2 tablespoons almond butter

- 3 sprigs of fresh thyme, chopped

- 3 eggs, beaten

- 1 tablespoon honey

- 2 tablespoons coconut oil

Directions:

1. In a bowl, mix together zucchini, apple, thyme, honey, and almond butter.

2. In a separate bowl, combine flour, iodized salt, and baking powder. Combine these ingredients with the wet ingredients and add the beaten eggs.

3. In a skillet, heat the coconut oil. Fry the pancakes until golden-brown on each side. Serve with yogurt and fresh fruit.

Mushroom Leek Stir-Fry

This is a super easy recipe that is not only delicious, but high in protein.

You will need:

*   3 cups shitake mushrooms

*   1 cup bean sprouts

*   1 onion, diced

*   2 leeks, sliced

*   3 cloves garlic, minced

*   1 knob of ginger, minced

*   1 teaspoon cumin

*   1 carrot, sliced

*   5 ounce rice noodles

- ½ cup tamari

- ½ teaspoon chili flakes

- 1 tablespoon coconut oil

Directions:

1. Cook the rice noodles according to the instructions on the package. Set aside in cold water.

2. Heat coconut oil in a pan and toast cumin until fragrant. Add onion, garlic, and ginger, and sauté for 3 minutes. Add leeks, mushrooms, carrot, and bean sprouts. Stir-fry until the mushrooms are soft.

3. Add tamari and chili, followed by the rice noodles. Cook for 2 more minutes, stirring to coat the noodles with the sauce. Serve immediately.

Roasted Sweet Potato Wedges

Try this delicious alternative to French fries. Sweet potatoes are an excellent source of vitamin A and vitamin B6.

You will need:

- 4 medium sweet potatoes, cut into wedges

- 2 tablespoons coconut oil

- A pinch of pepper flakes

- Sea salt and pepper to taste

- Optional additions: thyme, cumin, oregano, or tarragon

Directions:

1. Preheat the oven to 425-degrees Fahrenheit.

2. Toss the sweet potato wedges with the coconut oil, sea salt, pepper, and any additional herbs you decide to use. Then, arrange them on a baking sheet.

3. Bake the sweet potato wedges for 45 minutes, turning them twice. Leaving the oven door slightly ajar enables the wedges to get crispy.

Braised Green Cabbage

Green cabbage promotes thyroid health. This braised recipe is mouth-watering and so simple. Keep in mind that cabbages contain goitrogens, therefore, they must always be cooked in order to inactivate the goitrogens in them.

You will need:

- 1 medium head of cabbage, cut into wedges

- 1 large yellow onion, cut into strips

- 1 large carrot, chopped

- ¼ cup chicken stock

- ¼ cup olive oil

- 1/8 teaspoon chili flakes

- Pepper and iodized salt to taste

Directions:

1. Heat the oven to 325-degrees Fahrenheit.

2. Arrange the cabbage wedges in a shallow baking pan. Scatter the onions and carrots atop the wedges.

3. Pour the chicken stock into the baking pan. Drizzle with olive oil and sprinkle with chili flakes, salt and pepper.

4. Cover and bake for 1 ½ hours, or until the cabbage is very tender. Remove the cover and bake for an additional 15 minutes to crisp the cabbage.

Goji Grapefruit Parsley Smoothie

Everyone loves smoothies. Here is a smoothie recipe that is easy to whip up and promotes thyroid health. Goji berries are a rich source of iron, selenium, vitamin C, and vitamin B2.

You will need:

-   1/3 cup goji berries

-   ½ grapefruit

-   A handful of fresh parsley

-   A handful of hemp seeds

-   1 ½ tablespoons ground flaxseed

-   1 tablespoon milk thistle

-   ¼ cup almonds, pecans, or walnuts

- 1 cup cold filtered water

Directions:

1. Combine all the ingredients in a blender. Blend until smooth.

Lima Bean Hummus

Lima beans are known to help stabilize blood sugar levels in patients suffering from thyroid disorders.

You will need:

- 1 can of lima beans

- The juice of 2 lemons

- 1 clove garlic, minced

- ½ teaspoon ground cumin

- ¼ cup fresh parsley, finely minced

- 1 tablespoon paprika

- Iodized salt to taste

Directions:

1. Simply blend all the ingredients—excluding the parsley—until pureed.

2. Transfer the hummus into a bowl and add the parsley. Refrigerate until chilled. Serve with chopped vegetables.

Banana Nut Bread

Bananas promote thyroid function as they are iodine-rich. Brazil nuts are a good source of selenium.

You will need:

- 2 ripe bananas, mashed

- 1 ½ cups brown rice flour

- 1 teaspoon baking powder

- ¾ cup cooked brown rice

- 3 egg whites, beaten

- ½ cup raisins

- 1/3 cup applesauce

- 1/3 cup Brazil nuts, coarsely chopped

- 1 teaspoon cinnamon

- ½ teaspoon pure vanilla extract

Directions:

1. Preheat oven to 350-degrees Fahrenheit.

2. In a bowl, combine the mashed bananas, applesauce, eggs, and vanilla.

3. In a separate bowl, combine the remaining dry ingredients. Add this mixture to the wet ingredients and combine well.

4. Pour the mixture into a greased loaf pan. Bake until the top is brown and a toothpick comes out clean.

Almond Flax-Coated Chicken

Here is a recipe that is both tasty and nutritious. It incorporates flaxseed, which contains polyunsaturated fats—a type of healthy fat.

You will need:

- 4 boneless, skinless chicken breasts

- 3 tablespoons ground flaxseed

- ½ cup almond meal

- 1 tablespoon extra-virgin olive oil

- 1 tablespoon almond butter

- 1 tablespoon yellow onion, finely chopped

- 1 teaspoon lemon juice

- 1 teaspoon sea salt

- 1/8 teaspoon cayenne pepper

- ¼ teaspoon paprika

- 1 teaspoon fresh parsley, chopped

- 1 teaspoon fresh thyme, chopped

Directions:

1. Preheat oven to 350-degrees Fahrenheit.

2. Pound the chicken breasts with a kitchen mallet until they are 1/2-inch thick.

3. In a small bowl, mix together flaxseed and almond meal.

4. In another bowl, combine the remaining ingredients. Add the chicken breasts to this mixture and toss until evenly coated. Marinate for at least half an hour.

5. Sprinkle half of the almond/flax crust over the tops of the chicken breasts and gently press the crust into each piece until evenly coated. Carefully turn the chicken over and repeat the process with the remaining almond and flax mixture.

6. Put the baking sheet into the oven on the top rack and bake until the juices run clear, 20 to 30 minutes. Any leftover chicken can be refrigerated for up to 3 days.

Conclusion

Thank you again for downloading this book!

I hope this book was able to help you learn more about improving thyroid disorders with diet! Simply put the steps provided into place and begin improving your thyroid function now! Remember to consult a medical professional when making dietary changes, and before seeking any thyroid disorder treatments.

Finally, if you enjoyed this book, please take the time to share your thoughts and post a review on Amazon. It'd be greatly appreciated!

Thank you and good luck!